Table of Contents

INTRODUCTION

Hair loss (alopecia) is a fairly common occurrence. While it's more prevalent in older adults, anyone can experience it, including children. It's typical to lose between 50 and 100 hairs a day, according to the American Academy of Dermatology (AAD). With about 100,000 hairs on your head, that small loss isn't noticeable. New hair normally replaces the lost hair, but this doesn't always happen. Hair loss can develop gradually over years or happen abruptly. Depending on the underlying cause, it may be temporary or permanent. Trying to tell if you're actually losing hair or just experiencing some normal shedding? Unsure if it's time to see a doctor? Read on for more information about hair loss and how to manage it.

Hair loss symptoms

The main symptom of alopecia is losing more hair than usual, but this can be harder to identify than you might think. The following symptoms can provide some clues:

Widening part. If you part your hair, you might start to notice your part getting wider, which can be a sign of thinning hair.

Receding hairline. Similarly, if you notice your hairline looking higher than usual, it may be a sign of thinning hair.

Loose hair. Check your brush or comb after using it. Is it collecting more hair than usual? If so, this may be a sign of hair loss.

Bald patches. These can range in size and can grow over time.

Clogged drains. You might find that your sink or shower drains are clogged with hair.

Pain or itching. If you have an underlying skin condition causing your hair loss, you might also feel pain or experience itching on your scalp.

What causes hair loss?

There are several types of hair loss, some are common and some are rarer, and each with different underlying causes. Depending on the type of hair loss, it can be the result of genetics, internal causes, or external causes. Here's a look at a few different types of hair loss:

Androgenic alopecia

Androgenic alopecia refers to hereditary hair loss, like male pattern baldness or female pattern baldness, and is also known as "pattern alopecia" because it can happen to both males and females. It's also the most common cause of hair loss, affecting up to 50% of peopleTrusted Source.

Alopecia areata

Alopecia areata is an autoimmune condition that causes your immune system to attack hair follicles, resulting in bald patches that can range from small to large. In some cases, it might lead to total hair loss. In addition to losing hair on the scalp, some people with alopecia areata lose hair from their eyebrows, eyelashes, or other parts of the body.

Anagen effluvium

Anagen effluvium involves a rapid loss of hair. This usually happens because of radiation treatment or chemotherapy. Hair will usually regrow after the treatment stops.

Telogen effluvium

Telogen effluvium is a type of sudden hair loss that results from emotional or physical shock, like a traumatic event, period of extreme stress, or a serious illness. It can also happen because of hormonal changes, like those that happen in:

childbirth

postpartum

menopause

Polycystic Ovary Syndrome (PCOS)

Other potential causes of telogen effluvium include:

malnutrition including vitamin or mineral deficiency

certain endocrine disorders

starting or stopping hormonal birth control

post surgery as a result of the anesthesia

acute illnesses or severe infections like COVID-19

Several types of medications can also cause it, including:

anticoagulants

anticonvulsants

oral retinoids

beta-blockers

thyroid medications

This type of hair loss typically resolves on its own once the underlying cause is addressed.

Tinea capitis

Tinea capitis, also called ringworm of the scalp, is a fungal infection that can affect the scalp and hair shaft. It causes small bald patches that are scaly and itchy. Over time, if not treated early, the size of the patch or patches will increase and fill with pus. These patches, sometimes called a kerion, can cause scarring as well. Other symptoms include:

brittle hair that breaks easily

scalp tenderness

scaly patches of skin that look grey or red

It's treatable with antifungal medication.

Traction alopecia

Traction alopecia results from too much pressure and tension on the hair, often from wearing it in tight styles, like braids, ponytails, or buns.

How is hair loss diagnosed?

Because so many things can cause hair loss, it's best to schedule an appointment with a medical professional if you notice any changes in your hair. They'll likely use a combination of your health history — including any recent illnesses, surgeries, life stressors, and family history — and a physical exam to help narrow down the causes.

If they suspect an autoimmune or skin condition, they might take a biopsy of the skin on your scalp. This involves carefully removing several small sections of skin for laboratory testing. It's important to keep in mind that hair growth is a complex process and multiple tests may be needed to understand what is causing your hair loss. A biopsy may also be taken if it is initially very unclear what the root causes may be. They may also order blood tests to check for any nutrient deficiencies or signs of an underlying condition.

What are the treatment options for hair loss?
There's a range of treatment options for hair loss, but the best option for you will depend on what's causing your hair loss. Typically, the most common types of hair loss are treated with topical or oral medications, which will likely be the first course of treatment. Over-the-counter (OTC) medications generally consist of topical creams, gels, solutions, or foams that you apply directly to the scalp. The most common products contain an ingredient called minoxidil.

Prescription medications, like finasteride (Propecia), may help prevent further androgenetic hair loss, especially for male pattern baldness. You take this medication daily to slow hair loss, though some experience new hair growth when taking finasteride. Your clinician might prescribe anti-inflammatory medications, like corticosteroids, if hair loss seems related to an autoimmune condition. Newer treatments that are also being explored include some forms of laser therapy, microneedling with PRP, as well as other oral medications. Many of these treatments are still in the early testing phases though, and more research will be necessary.

Hair transplant surgery

Hair transplant surgery involves moving small plugs of skin, each with a few hairs, to bald parts of your scalp. This works well for people with inherited baldness since they typically lose hair on the top of the head. Because some hair loss can be progressive, you may need multiple procedures over time. It is worth noting that this method is unlikely to benefit or help people with scarring alopecias.

How can I prevent hair loss?

There are a few things you can do to minimize hair loss:

Keep hairstyles loose. If you regularly style your hair into braids, buns, or ponytails, try to keep them loose so they don't put too much pressure on your hair.

Avoid touching your hair. As much as possible, try not to pull, twist, or rub your hair.

Pat hair dry. After washing, use a towel to gently pat your hair dry. Avoid rubbing your hair with the towel or twisting it within the towel.

Aim for a nutrient-rich balanced diet. Try to incorporate plenty of iron and protein into snacks and meals.

Styling products and tools are also common culprits in hair loss. Examples of products or tools that can affect hair loss include:

blow dryers

heated combs

hair straighteners

coloring products

bleaching agents

perms

relaxers

If you decide to style your hair with heated tools, only do so when your hair is dry and use the lowest settings possible. If you're currently losing hair, use a gentle baby shampoo to wash your hair. Unless you have extremely oily hair, consider washing your hair only every other day or less.

When to see a doctor about hair loss

It's best to see a healthcare professional for any unexplained hair loss so they can determine the underlying cause and best course of treatment. During your appointment, be sure to mention any other unusual symptoms you've noticed, including:

fatigue

unexplained weight loss

fever

changes in bowel movements

rashes or other skin changes on your scalp or body

recent surgeries or medical procedures

changes to your diet and nutrition

any new immunizations or medications

Any information you can provide about how quickly the hair loss occurred, along with any family history of baldness, will also be helpful. If you need help finding a primary care doctor, then check out our FindCare tool here.

Frequently asked questions about hair loss

Which vitamin can help with hair loss?

Hair loss is a complicated topic and the role of nutrition in preventing or treating hair loss can be somewhat controversial. While nutrition and specific nutrients are vital to the hair growth process, increasing your intake of these nutrients may not help you, especially if you have a certain type of hair loss, such as scarring alopecia or cicatricial alopecia. Vitamins to incorporate into your nutrition plan that may promote hair growth include:

B vitamins, specifically riboflavin, biotin, folate, and vitamin B12 iron

vitamin C

vitamin D

Some researchTrusted Source connects excess intake of vitamin A or selenium with an increased risks for hair loss.

What illness causes hair loss?
An increased risk of hair loss is connected with certain illnesses. These include:

polycystic ovary syndrome (PCOS)

scalp psoriasis

sexually transmitted infections, such as syphilis

thyroid disease

Hair loss can also be a side effect of some medications, especially chemotherapy medications to treat cancers.

Is it possible to stop hair loss indefinitely?
Stopping hair loss indefinitely depends upon the underlying cause. As a general rule, the sooner you treat hair loss, the

more likely you will be able to reverse or reduce the rate of hair loss. Some hair loss causes can't be reversed. This is true for damaged hair follicles from too-tight hairstyles, damaged hair follicles from chemicals applied to the hair, and damages caused by certain autoimmune diseases.

Whatever the cause of your hair loss, seeking medical attention from your primary care doctor or a dermatologist can help you identify underlying causes. Treatments for hair loss are more likely to be successful if started early. Treatments may include changes to how you care for your hair, improvements to your diet, and medical treatments that may be topically applied or taken in orally. Even if your hair loss is hereditary, there are treatments that exist that can help slow or reverse hair loss. If possible, talk with your doctor to address your concerns and rule out any serious underlying medical concerns that may be causing your hair loss.

Does Stress Cause Hair Loss?

Hair loss is clinically known as alopecia. Both men and women may experience hair loss in their lifetime. If you're experiencing hair loss, it may be caused by stress. Keep reading to learn how stress can affect your hair health, whether its effects are permanent, and what you can do to help encourage regrowth.

Types of stress-related hair loss

Not all hair loss is caused by stress. There are three types of hair loss that are associated with high stress levels:

Telogen effluvium

Telogen effluvium (TE) occurs when there's a change to the number of hair follicles that are actually growing hair. If this change occurs during the telogen — or resting — phase of hair growth, it can result in shedding. This thinning may not occur all over the head. It's often seen in patches, especially toward the center of the scalp. People affected by TE usually don't lose all of their scalp hair. In more extreme cases, you may experience thinning hair on other parts of the body. This includes the eyebrows or the genital area.

TE may be the second most common type of hair loss seen by dermatologists. It can happen to men and women at any age. The hair loss that occurs from TE is fully reversible. TE doesn't permanently damage the hair follicles. The cause of your TE will affect whether your hair grows back in a few short months, or longer.

Alopecia areata

Alopecia areata (AA) is an autoimmune disease. It develops when your immune system attacks your hair follicles. This may be triggered by stress, and it can result in hair loss..Hair may be lost in round patches on the scalp, or across the entire scalp. In a more severe form of AA known as alopecia universalis, hair is lost from the entire body.

The hair may grow back and fall out repeatedly over a period of time. AA can affect men and women of any age, affecting over six million people in the United States. There is no known cure for AA, though there are some prescription medications that may help those with over 50 percent hair loss.

Trichotillomania

Trichotillomania is also known as hair pulling disorder. It involves the urge to pull out the hair from your scalp or other parts of your body. It's considered an impulse control disorder. You may find that hair pulling happens without much thought, like when you're bored or distracted. The hair pulling may also be more intentional and used as a means to relieve stress or other negative emotions. Hair pulling from the scalp, eyebrows, and eyelashes is often noticeable. This may cause additional stress, perpetuating the cycle of the disorder.

Trichotillomania most often develops in preteens, and can last a lifetime. Although it isn't clear what causes trichotillomania, research suggests that it may be genetic.

Is stress-related hair loss permanent?

If your hair loss is caused by stress, it's possible for your hair to grow back in time. The rate of regrowth will be different for everyone. Human hair growth occurs in a cycle of four phases.

The average human scalp has about 100,000 hair follicles. At any given time, each of your hair follicles is in a different phase of this cycle:

Anagen phase. This is the growing phase of hair. It lasts two to seven years

Catagen phase. This is a short, two-week phase that occurs when the hair follicle begins to shrink.

Telogen phase. This is a three-month resting phase.

Exogen phase. This phase occurs when the follicle sheds the hair and begins new growth.

If your hair loss has been triggered by stress, managing your stress could be the key to returning to a healthy rate of hair growth.

What you can do

There are a number of things that you can do to reduce hair loss and encourage new growth.

Diet and nutrition

Eating a balanced, nutritious diet of whole foods is necessary for the health of your body — and your hair.

While it's important to include all of the essential vitamins in a healthy diet, there are some that may be vital to hair growth:

Vitamin C.This vitaminis essential for building collagen, the skin's connective tissue that is found in hair follicles. Foods that contain vitamin C include citrus fruits, broccoli, bell peppers, and strawberries.

Vitamin B. This complex of many vitamins promotes a healthy metabolism, as well as healthy skin and hair. B vitamins can be found in foods like dark leafy greens, beans, nuts, and avocados.

Vitamin E.This vitamin contains potent antioxidants, which can contribute to a healthy scalp. Foods rich in vitamin E include sunflower seeds, spinach, olive oil, broccoli, and shrimp.

If you aren't getting enough of these nutrients in your diet, talk to your doctor about supplements. They can discuss your options and recommend the best dosage for you. You should never add nutritional supplements to your routine without your doctor's supervision.

Keeping properly hydrated is also essential to overall good health. Every cell in your body relies on water to function properly. Men should aim for 15 1/2 cups of water per day, and women should aim for 11 1/2 cups per day. That amount can come from food, water, and other beverages. A reasonable goal is to drink 8 glasses of water per day, and allow the rest to come from your diet and other beverages.

Stress management

Learning how to effectively manage your stress levels may help you reduce your risk for further hair loss. Of course, this is often easier said than done. You may have to try several different stress-management techniques before you find what works for you.

Popular ways to reduce stress:

Exercise. Exercise is a great way to eliminate stress. Try taking a light daily walk, signing up for a dance class, or doing some yard work.

Hobbies. Occupying yourself with something that you enjoy doing can be a great way to combat stress. Consider doing volunteer work, joining your local community theatre group, planting a garden, or starting an art project.

Writing. Try taking a few minutes each day to write about your feelings, and the things that cause you stress. Reviewing the daily items that trigger your stress may help you to discover ways of coping with it.

Breathing and meditation. Meditation and breathing exercises are great ways to allow yourself to focus on the present moment. You may also wish to try techniques that combine meditation with physical exercise, like yoga or tai chi.

Topical treatments

There are a number of topical creams, oils, and other products that may help with your hair loss.

Topical Minoxidil (Rogaine). Topical minoxidil is an over-the-counter (OTC) medication. It's available as a cream, spray, or foam. You can apply it to your scalp, eyebrows, or beard up to twice daily. It isn't appropriate for other parts of the body. There are variations formulated specifically for male or female use. Although it isn't clear how minoxidil works, it's thought to prolong the growth phase. It may not work for everyone, and results may take up to four months to see.

Topical corticosteroids. Topical OTC and prescription corticosteroids, like prednisone, are sometimes used to treat alopecia areata. They're often used alongside other treatment options.

Castor oil. This is a popular folk remedy for hair regrowth. Although anecdotal evidence suggests that topical use can increase hair growth, research to support this is limited.Trusted Source

What if you aren't seeing improvement?

It's possible that your hair loss isn't stress related. There are many factors and conditions that could cause you to lose your hair.Other common reasons for hair loss include:

aging

genetics

medications, like some blood thinners or antidepressants

chemotherapy

illness or recent surgery

hormonal changes, like childbirth or menopause

nutritional deficiency, like a lack of sufficient protein or iron

If your hair loss is stress related, your hair follicles haven't been permanently damaged. Managing your stress and taking good care of your health could result in your hair returning to a normal rate of growth.

If OTC measures aren't working — or you aren't seeing results — see your doctor. They can help diagnose the reason for your hair loss and advise you on any next steps. If regrowth is possible, they can help determine the best treatment plan for your symptoms.

WHAT IS MALE PATTERN BALDNESS?

Male pattern baldness, also called androgenic alopecia, is the most common type of hair loss in men. According to the U.S. National Library of Medicine (NLM), more than 50 percent of all men over the age of 50 will be affected by male pattern baldness to some extent

What causes male pattern baldness?

One cause of male pattern baldness is genetics, or having a family history of baldness. Research has found that male pattern baldness is associated with male sex hormones called androgens. The androgens have many functions, including regulating hair growth. Each hair on your head has a growth cycle. With male pattern baldness, this growth cycle begins to weaken and the hair follicle shrinks, producing shorter and finer strands of hair. Eventually, the growth cycle for each hair ends and no new hair grows in its place. Inherited male pattern baldness usually has no side effects. However, sometimes baldness has more serious causes, such as certain cancers, medications, thyroid conditions, and anabolic steroids. See your doctor if hair loss occurs after taking new medications or when it's accompanied by other health complaints.

Doctors use the pattern of hair loss to diagnose male pattern baldness. They may perform a medical history and exam to rule out certain health conditions as the cause, such as fungal conditions of the scalp or nutritional disorders. Health conditions may be a cause of baldness when a rash, redness, pain, peeling of the scalp, hair breakage, patchy hair loss, or an unusual pattern of hair loss accompanies the hair loss. A skin biopsy and blood tests also may be necessary to diagnose disorders responsible for the hair loss.

Who's at risk?

Male pattern baldness can begin in your teenage years, but it more commonly occurs in adult men, with the likelihood increasing with age. Genetics plays a big role. Men who have close relatives with male pattern baldness are at a higher risk. This is particularly true when their relatives are on the maternal side of the family.

Am I losing my hair?

If your hair loss begins at the temples or the crown of the head, you may have male pattern baldness. Some men will get a single bald spot. Others experience their hairlines receding to form an "M" shape. In some men, the hairline will continue to recede until all or most of the hair is gone.

Techniques to address hair loss

Medical treatment isn't necessary if other health conditions aren't a cause. However, treatments are available for men who are unhappy with the way they look and would like the appearance of a fuller head of hair.

Hairstyles

Men with limited hair loss can sometimes hide hair loss with the right haircut or hairstyle. Ask your hairstylist for a creative cut that will make thinning hair look fuller.

Wigs or hairpieces

Wigs can cover thinning hair, receding hairlines, and complete baldness. They come in a variety of styles, colors, and textures. For a natural look, choose wig colors, styles, and textures that look similar to your original hair. Professional wig stylists can help style and fit wigs for an even more natural look.

Weaves

Hair weaves are wigs that are sewn into your natural hair. You must have enough hair to sew the weave into. The advantage to weaves is they always stay on, even during activities such as swimming, showering, and sleeping. The disadvantages are they must be sewn again whenever new hair growth occurs, and the sewing process can damage your natural hair.

Minoxidil (Rogaine)

Minoxidil (Rogaine) is a topical medication applied to the scalp. Minoxidil slows hair loss for some men and stimulates the hair follicles to grow new hair. Minoxidil takes four months to one year to produce visible results. Hair loss often happens again when you stop taking the medication. Possible side effects associated with minoxidil include dryness, irritation, burning, and scaling of the scalp. You should visit the doctor immediately if you have any of these serious side effects:

weight gain

swelling of the face, hands, ankles, or abdomen

trouble breathing when lying down

rapid heartbeat

chest pain

labored respiration

Finasteride (Propecia, Proscar)

Finasteride (Propecia, Proscar) is an oral medication that slows hair loss in some men. It works by blocking the production of the male hormone responsible for hair loss. Finasteride has a higher success rate than minoxidil. When you stop taking finasteride, your hair loss returns. You must take finasteride for three months to one year before you see results. If no hair growth occurs after one year, your doctor will likely recommend that you stop taking the medication. The side effects of finasteride include:

depression

itching

rash

hives

breast tenderness

breast growth

swelling of the face or lips

painful ejaculation

pain in testicles

difficulty getting an erection

Although it's rare, finasteride can cause breast cancer. You should have any breast pain or lumps evaluated by a doctor immediately. Finasteride may affect prostate-specific antigen (PSA) tests used to screen for prostate cancer. The medication lowers PSA levels, which causes lower-than-normal readings. Any rise in PSA levels when taking finasteride should be evaluated for prostate cancer.

Hair transplants

A hair transplant is the most invasive and expensive treatment for hair loss. Hair transplants work by removing hair from areas of the scalp that have active hair growth and transplanting them to thinning or balding areas of your scalp. Multiple treatments are often necessary, and the procedure carries the risk of scarring and infection. The advantages of a hair transplant are that it looks more natural and it's permanent.

Counseling

Going bald can be a big change. You may have trouble accepting your appearance. You should seek counseling if you experience anxiety, low self-esteem, depression, or other emotional problems because of male pattern baldness.

Can hair loss be prevented?

There's no known way to prevent male pattern baldness. A theory is that stress may cause hair loss by increasing the production levels of sex hormones in the body. You can reduce stress by participating in relaxing activities, such as walking, listening to calming music, and enjoying more quiet time.

What to Know About Female Hair Loss

Hair loss can be caused by many factors, including nutrient deficiencies, stress, certain health conditions, and changes in hormone levels. Early diagnosis and treatment may help stop hair loss and promote hair regrowth.

What is hair loss in AFAB folks?

Some degree of hair loss is healthy and unnoticeable — people lose around 50 to 100 hairs a day on average. But it can be more severe.In people assigned female at birth (AFAB), noticeable hair loss is pretty common, with around one third experiencing it at some point. However, whether it's subtle thinning all over or a bare patch where the scalp can be seen, it can look different to the typical "baldness" you might expect. And there are various types with various causes. For example, the thinning hair associated with female pattern baldness is different from the mass shedding of telogen effluvium.

What causes it?

From dietary deficiencies to stress, hair loss in AFAB folks can have a number of causes.Telogen effluvium — when significantly more hairs move from the growing to the shedding stage — can occur after a traumatic or stressful experience, such as:

childbirth

extreme weight loss,

the loss of a loved one

Deficiencies of vitamins, like vitamin DTrusted Source, and minerals, like iron, are believed to also contribute. They are needed to produce healthy strandsTrusted Source of hair. Triggers for other types of hair loss range from inflammatory scalp conditions, like eczema, to an underlying health concern, such as an autoimmune condition. Even tight hairstyles, like ponytails or braids, can lead to hair loss as a result of putting pressure on roots.

What is female pattern baldness?

Female pattern baldness — also known as androgenetic alopecia — is hair loss that affects people assigned female at birth. It's similar to male pattern baldness, except that the hair loss tends to occur in a different pattern.

What causes female pattern baldness?

Female pattern baldness is usually hereditary — caused by a genetically shorter hair-growing period and a longer period between the shedding and growth phases. Genes from parents may also affect the hair, causing smaller follicles and thinner strands. However, age and hormones may play a part, too, as it's more common after menopause when estrogen levels reduce.

This means that the effects of male androgen hormones — which are linked to male pattern baldness —may be greater. More androgenetic activity can also occur through an underlying endocrine condition, such as a tumor on the ovary gland.

What does female pattern baldness look like?

In female pattern baldness, the hair's growing phase slows down. It also takes longer for new hair to begin growing. Hair follicles shrink, leading the hair that does grow to be thinner and finer. This can result in hair that easily breaks.People with this condition also tend to shed more hairs than the average person, though complete baldness is less likely. In male pattern baldness, hair loss starts in the front of the head and recedes to the back until the person goes bald. But female pattern baldness starts at the part line, sometimes appearing all over the head. Hair at the temples may also recede. Doctors divide the condition into three types:

Type I is a small amount of thinning that starts around the part.

Type II involves widening of the part and increased thinning around it.

Type III is thinning throughout, with a see-through area at the top of the scalp.

Treatment for female pattern baldness

If you have female pattern baldness, you may be able to camouflage the hair loss at first by adopting a new hairstyle.

But it often becomes too difficult to hide the thinning hair. Early diagnosis is encouraged, as it can enable you to start a treatment plan and potentially minimize future hair loss. Your treatment plan will likely consist of one or more medications approved to treat the condition.

Minoxidil

Minoxidil (Rogaine) is the only drug approved by the Food and Drug Administration (FDA) to treat female pattern baldness. It's available in 2% or 5% formulas. If possible, opt for the 5% formula — older studiesTrusted Source found that it's superior. Apply minoxidil to your scalp every day. Though it won't fully restore the hair you've lost, it can grow back a significant amount of hairTrusted Source and give an overall thicker appearance. It can take around 6 to 12 months to see results. And you'll need to keep using minoxidil to maintain the effect, or it'll stop working. If this happens, your hair may return to its previous appearance.

The following side effects are possible:

redness

dryness

itching

hair growth on areas where you didn't want it, such as your cheeks

Finasteride and dutasteride

Finasteride (Propecia) and dutasteride (Avodart) are FDA approved to treat male pattern hair loss. They're not approved for female pattern hair loss, but some doctors do recommend them. Studies are mixed about the effectiveness of these drugs for AFAB folks, but some researchTrusted Source shows that they do help regrow hair in female pattern baldness. Side effects can include:

headaches

hot flashes

decreased sex drive, especially during the first year of use

People also should avoid becoming pregnant, because it can increase the risk for birth defects.

Spironolactone

Spironolactone (Aldactone) is a diuretic, which means it removes excess fluid from the body. It also blocks androgen production and therefore may help regrow hair that's been lost as a result of female pattern baldness. This medication can cause a number of side effects, including:

electrolyte imbalances

fatigue

spotting between periods

irregular menstruation

tender breasts

You may need to have regular blood pressure and electrolyte tests while you take it. If you're pregnant or plan to become pregnant, you shouldn't use this medication due to the risk of birth defects.

Other options

Laser combs and helmets are also FDA approved to treat hair loss. They use light energy to stimulate hair regrowth, but more research needs to be done to determine if this is truly effective. Platelet-rich plasma therapy may also be beneficial. This involves drawing your blood, spinning it down, then injecting your own platelets back into your scalp to stimulate hair growth. Though promising, more studies need to be done. Similarly, there isn't any evidence that taking iron will regrow your hair. But if low iron is contributing to your hair loss, a doctor or other healthcare professional still might prescribe an iron supplement. Other supplements, such as biotin and folic acid, are also promoted to thicken hair.

A 2015 study showed that people developed thicker hair after taking omega-3 fatty acids, omega-6 fatty acids, and antioxidants. However, it's best to check with a healthcare professional before taking any supplements with this aim. If you want a simple way to conceal hair loss, you might try a wig or spray hair product. A hair transplant is a more permanent solution. During this procedure, a healthcare professional removes a thin strip of hair from one part of your scalp and implants it in an area where you're missing hair. The graft regrows like your natural hair.

How is it diagnosed?

A doctor or dermatologist can give a diagnosis for thinning hair. Testing generally isn't necessary, but they'll examine your scalp to see the pattern of hair loss. If they suspect another type of hair loss other than female pattern baldness, they may also perform a blood test to check your levels of thyroid hormone, androgens, iron, or other substances that can affect hair growth.

Can genetics cause female pattern baldness?

Hair loss is passed down from biological parents to their children, and many genes are involved. You can inherit these genes from either biological parent. You're more likely to develop female pattern baldness if your biological parents or other close genetic relatives have experienced hair loss.

What else causes female pattern baldness?

Female pattern baldness is generally caused by an underlying endocrine condition or a hormone-secreting tumor. You could consult a healthcare professional if you have other symptoms, such as:

irregular period

severe acne

increase in unwanted hair

These may be a sign that you're experiencing a different type of hair loss.

Can people get female pattern baldness in their 20s?

People are less likely to develop female pattern baldness before midlife and are more likely to start losing hair once they get into their 40s, 50s, and beyond.

Is it reversible?

While some forms of AFAB hair loss are temporary, female pattern baldness is permanent and irreversible without treatment. However, proper treatment can stop the hair loss and potentially help regrow some lost hair. You'll need to stay on this treatment long-term to prevent losing your hair again.

Can female pattern baldness worsen?

Female pattern baldness will progressTrusted Source without treatment. However, progression is often slow, taking years to even decades to worsen. You might notice periods of stability followed by more rapid hair loss phases. And the earlier you experience female pattern baldness, the quicker it may progress.

Can you prevent female pattern baldness?

You can't prevent it, but you can protect your hair from breakage and loss via the following:

Hair care tips

Eat a balanced diet. Get enough iron from foods, like dark green leafy vegetables, beans, and fortified cereals.

Limit treatments that can break or damage your hair, such as straightening irons, bleach, and perms. If you do use them, add a heat protective spray or hair-strengthening product to your routine.

Ask a healthcare professional if any of the medications you take promote hair loss. If so, see if you can switch.

Limit or quit smoking. It damages hair follicles and can speed up hair loss.

Wear a hat or carry a parasol when you go outside. Too much sun exposure can damage hair.

If you're noticing hair loss, consider reaching out to a doctor or dermatologist. They'll be able to figure out what kind of hair loss it is and what could potentially be causing it. Plus, they'll be able to recommend and prescribe the best form of treatment. The sooner you receive treatment, the faster you'll be able to stop the loss — and possibly even regrow some of your hair.

Laser Treatment for Hair Loss

Every day, most people lose about 100 hairs from their scalp. While the majority of people grow those hairs grow back, some people don't due to:

age

heredity

hormonal changes

medical conditions, such as lupus and diabetes

poor nutrition

side effects of a medical treatment, such as chemotherapy

stress

Treatments to stop hair loss and possibly reverse it include:

medications such as minoxidil (Rogaine) and finasteride (Propecia)

hair transplant surgery

laser therapy

Does laser treatment for hair loss work?

What it does

Low-level laser therapy — also referred to as red light therapy and cold laser therapy — irradiates photons into scalp tissues. These photons are absorbed by weak cells to encourage hair growth.

It's widely accepted that the procedure is safe, tolerable, and less invasive than hair transplant surgery.

The theory

The theory of laser treatment for hair loss is that the low-dose laser treatments invigorate circulation and stimulation that encourages hair follicles to grow hair.

The results

Because the results of laser therapy are inconsistent, the conclusion of the medical community seems to be that it appears to work for some people, but not for others. More research is needed, but some studies have yielded encouraging results:

According to a 2014 study low-level laser therapy appeared to be safe and effective for hair growth in both men and women.

A 2013 studyTrusted Source of 41 males ages 18 to 48 found that laser hair treatment provided a 39 percent increase in hair growth over a period of 16 weeks.

What are the positives of laser treatment for hair loss?

There are a number of reasons that advocates cite to encourage participation in the procedure, including:

it's noninvasive

it's painless

there are no side effects

it increases hair strength

What are the negatives of laser treatment for hair loss?

There are a number of reasons that some people are not as positive about the procedure, such as:

It's time consuming. To see results, treatment often requires several sessions a week for a number of months. Although the number of sessions might taper off, most providers suggest that you continue treatments for the rest of your life.

It's expensive. Clinical laser treatments for hair loss can cost thousands of dollars a year.

It may not be effective. The procedure appears to be less effective for people in the advanced stages of hair loss as opposed to those in the early stages.

It can interact with certain medications. Laser therapy should not be performed on people taking medications that are photosensitizing. Photosensitizing is a chemical alteration to the skin that increases someone's sensitivity to light.

Long-term safety and effectiveness have not yet been established. Laser devices are classified as medical devices by the FDA so they don't have the same level of scrutiny and testing that medicines go through prior to approval. Long-term safety and long-term effectiveness have not yet been established.

If you want to stop and perhaps reverse hair loss, you might consider laser treatment as an option. As with any treatment, there are some positives and negatives that should be considered when determining if it's right for you. Your doctor can help you make a good decision. If you lose hair suddenly, see your doctor. Rapid hair loss might be an indication of an underlying condition that needs to be addressed.

PRP for Hair Loss

PRP (platelet-rich plasma) therapy for hair loss is a three-step medical treatment in which a person's blood is drawn, processed, and then injected into the scalp. Some in the medical community think that PRP injections trigger natural hair growth and maintain it by increasing blood supply to the hair follicle and increasing the thickness of the hair shaft. Sometimes this approach is combined with other hair loss procedures or medications. There hasn't been enough research to prove if PRP is an effective hair loss treatment. However, PRP therapy has been in use since the 1980s. It's been used for problems such as healing injured tendons, ligaments, and muscles.

PRP therapy process

PRP therapy is a three-step process. Most PRP therapy requires three treatments 4–6 weeks apart. Maintenance treatments are required every 4–6 months.

Step 1

Your blood is drawn — typically from your arm — and put into a centrifuge (a machine that spins rapidly to separate fluids of different densities).

Step 2

After about 10 minutes in the centrifuge, your blood will have separated into in three layers:

platelet-poor plasma

platelet-rich plasma

red blood cells

Step 3

The platelet-rich plasma is drawn up into a syringe and then injected into areas of the scalp that need increased hair growth. There hasn't been enough research to prove whether PRP is effective. It's also unclear for whom — and under what circumstances — it's most effective. According to a recent studyTrusted Source, "Although PRP has sufficient theoretical scientific basis to support its use in hair restoration, hair restoration using PRP is still at its infancy. Clinical evidence is still weak."

PRP for hair loss side effects

Because PRP therapy involves injecting your own blood into your scalp, you aren't at risk for getting a communicable disease. Still, any therapy that involves injections always carries a risk of side effects such as:

injury to blood vessels or nerves

infection

calcification at the injection points

scar tissue

There's also the chance that you could have a negative reaction to the anesthetic used in the therapy. If you decide to pursue PRP therapy for hair loss, let your doctor know in advance about your tolerance to anesthetics.

Risks of PRP for hair loss

Be sure to report all medications you're on before the procedure including supplements and herbs. When you go for your initial consultation, many providers will recommend against PRP for hair loss if you:

are on blood thinners

are a heavy smoker

have a history of alcohol or drug misuse

You might also be rejected for treatment if you've been diagnosed with:

acute or chronic infections

cancer

chronic liver disease

chronic skin disease

hemodynamic instability

hypofibrinogenemia

metabolic disorder

platelet dysfunction syndromes

systemic disorder

sepsis

low platelet count

thyroid disease

How much does PRP for hair loss cost?

PRP therapy typically consists of three treatments in a 4–6 week period, with maintenance treatments every 4–6 months. The price typically ranges from $1,500–$3,500 for the initial three treatments, with one injection at $400 or more. Pricing depends on a number of factors including:

your geographic location

quality of equipment

the addition of nutritive components

Many insurance plans consider PRP for hair loss treatment to be cosmetic and don't cover any of the costs of the treatment. Check with your insurance provider to see if PRP therapy is covered for you.

If you're concerned about hair loss, you have a number of options including medication like Rogaine and Propecia, along with hair transplant surgery. Another consideration is PRP therapy. Although there's limited clinical proof that PRP for hair loss works, there are many who believe that PRP is a safe and effective way of reversing hair loss and stimulating new hair growth. Talk to your doctor to see which treatment or combination of treatments is the best choice for you.

12 WAYS TO STOP HAIR THINNING

You may be able to address thinning hair or bald spots with these 12 options. A doctor can also diagnose any underlying medical conditions and recommend medications to help..It's common to lose 50–100 hairs per day, according to the American Academy of Dermatology (AAD). Any more than this could mean you're shedding more than you should, which could contribute to overall thinning hair. Unlike widespread hair loss, thinning hair doesn't necessarily cause baldness. It does, however, give the appearance of sparser spots of hair on your head. Thinning hair typically happens gradually, which means you have time to pinpoint the causes and figure out the best treatment measures.

What causes thinning hair?

Thinning hair may be caused by lifestyle habits, genetics, or both. Certain medical conditions may also lead to thinning hair. Lifestyle habits may include:

Overtreating your hair: This includes color treatments, perms, and relaxers.

Using harsh hair products: These hair products include extreme-hold hair sprays and gels.

Wearing tight hairstyles: Whether you're wearing an updo or pulling your hair up in a ponytail for working out, this can tug on your hair and break it from the follicles, causing thin spots over time.

Not getting enough of certain nutrients in your diet: Iron, folic acid, and other minerals all help follicles produce hair naturally.

Experiencing chronic stress: Stress is related to an uptick in hormones like cortisol. Too many stress hormones can trigger a condition like telogen effluvium, in which your hair can fall out, and the hair follicles enter a long "resting" phase where new hair doesn't grow.

Thinning hair may also be hereditary or from underlying medical conditions. You might have thinning hair if you:

recently had a baby

recently stopped taking birth control pills

are going through hormonal changes

lost a significant amount of weight in a short amount of time

are being treated for an autoimmune disease

have immune system deficiencies

have a skin disorder or infection

have a vitamin D deficiency

are deficient in other vitamins and minerals like riboflavin, selenium, and zincTrusted Source

Less commonly, thinning hair may be caused by:

pulling at your own hair

eating disorders

a high fever

Hair thinning treatments and home remedies

Some cases of thinning hair may be treatable at home. Consider the following 12 options, but be sure to talk with your doctor first.

1. Scalp massage

Pros: It's affordable and accessible.

Cons: It doesn't address thinning hair caused by underlying medical conditions.

Perhaps the cheapest method of trying to get thicker hair is scalp massage. It doesn't cost anything, and if done correctly, it isn't harmful. When you wash your hair, gently apply pressure with your fingertips around your scalp to encourage blood flow. For even more benefits, you can try a handheld scalp massager to also remove dead skin cells.

2. Essential oils

Pros: Animal research suggests effectiveness, and essential oils are widely available in health shops and drugstores.

Cons: More human studies are needed, and these oils may cause allergic reactions.

Essential oils are liquids derived from certain plants, and they're primarily used in aromatherapy and other types of alternative medicine. Lavender oil has been used with success by some people with pattern baldness. It's also backed by animal research from 2016, though human studies are needed to confirm its effects. Lavender is often combined with other oils, such as those made from rosemary and thyme.

Still, there's not enough evidence that essential oils can treat baldness or thinning hair. If you do decide to give this treatment a go, make sure that your essential oil is diluted in a carrier oil such as coconut oil or jojoba). Test a small amount of the oil on your arm and wait 24 hours to see if any reaction develops. Redness or other irritation, hives, or a rash could indicate an allergic reaction. While research suggests there are health benefits, the FDA doesn't monitor or regulate the purity or quality of essential oils. It's important to talk with a healthcare professional before you begin using essential oils and be sure to research the quality of a brand's products. Always do a patch test before trying a new essential oil.

3. Anti-thinning shampoo

Pros: It can be combined with scalp massage, and some products are accessible over the counter.

Cons: Volumizing shampoos don't address hair loss alone, and you may require a prescription.

Anti-thinning shampoo works in two ways. First, such products provide volume for your hair, so it looks thicker. This can be helpful for people who have thinning or naturally fine hair. Shampoos for thinning hair or hair loss also contain vitamins and amino acids to promote a healthier scalp. To get the best results, use these products as directed.

4. Multivitamins

Pros: Multivitamins can help address thinning hair caused by nutritional deficiencies, and they're available over the counter.

Cons: Excess nutrients may be harmful.

Healthy hair is dependent on your overall good health. In cases of malnourishment or with certain eating disorders, new hair may fail to generate from follicles. A blood test can help determine if you have a nutrient deficiency. If you're low in several key areas, your doctor might recommend a daily multivitamin. Healthy hair needs iron, folic acid, and zinc to keep growing thick and strong. Look for daily supplements for males and females that meet these criteria.

However, you should avoid taking any extra vitamins if you're already getting the nutrients you need. There isn't any evidence that doing so will reverse thinning hair, and getting too much of certain nutrients may actually do more harm than good.

5. Folic acid supplements

Pros: These supplements are available over the counter and may treat folate deficiency.

Cons: There's a lack of evidence about their effectiveness.

Folic acid is a type of vitamin B that's important for new cell generation. A few studies have suggested that folate deficiency may be associated with some types of hair loss..But, as with multivitamins, there isn't enough evidence that folic acid is guaranteed to help make your hair thicker.

6. Biotin

Pros: Biotin is widely available over the counter, and may treat biotin deficiency.

Cons: There's not enough evidence that it helps with thinning hair.

Biotin, or vitamin B7, is a water-soluble nutrient that's naturally found in foods, such as nuts, lentils, and liver. If you eat a balanced diet, it's unlikely that you're low in biotin. However, supplemental forms of biotin have been on the rise in recent years, thanks in part to marketers promising more energy and better hair growth with such products.

While biotin helps break down enzymes in your body, there's little evidence that it can help with thinning hair. You shouldn't take biotin if you take vitamin B5 supplements. When taken together, they can reduce the efficacy of one another.

7. Omega-3 and omega-6 fatty acids

Pros: These fatty acids help fight inflammation, and these supplements are available over the counter.

Cons: More research is needed.

Omega-3 and omega-6 fatty acids are called essential fatty acids. This is because they can't be made by the human body. Omega-3 helps your body fight inflammation, an underlying cause of numerous conditions. Premature hair loss may also be related to inflammation. Omega-6, on the other hand, is important for overall skin health, which might benefit the scalp.

Plant-based oils are primary sources of omega-6, while omega-3 fatty acids are found in fish and some seeds. If you don't normally consume such foods, talk with your doctor about taking a supplement.

8. Minoxidil

Pros: Minoxidil is approved by the Food and Drug Administration (FDA), and it's available over the counter.

Cons: Scalp irritation is possible, and you must use it continuously to maintain results.

Best known by its brand name Rogaine, minoxidil is an over-the-counter hair loss treatment approved by the FDA..When applied directly to the scalp twice a day, minoxidil may gradually thicken hair in balding spots. The product is available in either liquid or foam, depending on your preference. It's also available as an oral prescription from your doctor. Rogaine can take up to 16 weeks for visible results. It's important that you use the product consistently, or you might not see results. Scalp irritation and unwanted hair growth on the face and neck are possible side effects.

9. Spironolactone

Pros: Spironolactone may treat thinning hair caused by excess aldosterone hormones.

Cons: It's available by prescription only and may cause headache, dizziness, and other side effects.

Spironolactone (Aldactone) is sometimes prescribed for people who have thinning hair related to aldosterone production (hyperaldosteronism). While technically a diuretic or "water pill," that may be prescribed for high blood pressure or edema, Aldactone is an anti-androgen, too. In females, this medication may help treat thinning hair and subsequent hair loss related to hormonal fluctuations.

10. Finasteride

Pros: This is the first FDA-approved oral medication for male hair loss.

Cons: It's available by prescription only and is generally not considered for females who are premenopausal.

Finasteride (Propecia) is a prescription hair loss medication. Unlike topical treatments like minoxidil, Propecia comes as a daily pill that males take for hair loss..People who are planning to become pregnant or are at an age where they may become pregnant should avoid this medication due to possible serious side effects during pregnancy. However, for postmenopausal females, studies have shown that it may be an effective treatment and is frequently prescribed by some doctors.

11. Corticosteroids

Pros: Corticosteroids help treat inflammation and autoimmune-related hair loss.

Cons: It's available by prescription only and long-term use may cause thinning skin and other side effects.

Corticosteroids are prescription treatments used for conditions linked to underlying inflammation. Sometimes, inflammatory conditions can cause a variety of symptoms, including hair loss. One example is alopecia areata, which is an autoimmune disorder where your immune system attacks hair follicles, causing thinning hair and sudden hair loss. Depending on the severity, hair loss may be mild or patchy, or more significant.

Prescription corticosteroids may help in these cases by controlling inflammation directly at the source: your hair follicles. Depending on the severity of hair loss, corticosteroids may be applied either topically or injected directly into the scalp by a dermatologist every 4–8 weeks.

12. At-home laser therapy

Pros: It's available without a prescription and can be used easily at home.

Cons: At-home laser therapy can be pricey, and it may also take several months to work.

Laser therapy is typically used by dermatologists and other skin specialists. The FDA has cleared the way for some products to be used at home. At-home laser therapy for hair is intended to help regrow your hair while also making it thicker. The results can take several months to take effect. The biggest drawback of at-home laser therapy is the cost. Some machines are sold for hundreds of dollars, and they may not work. Talk with your doctor before making a large investment.

Hair loss prevention tips

If you have an underlying medical condition, such as alopecia areata, getting the correct treatments from your doctor may help with hair loss. But, if a doctor doesn't believe your hair loss is related to a medical cause, there may be steps you can take to help prevent future hair loss. Consider the following:

Try to eat a balanced diet

Hair loss may be associated with a lack of micronutrients, such as iron, as well as macronutrients like protein. If you need help with meal planning, consider talking with a doctor or dietitian..It's also a good idea to talk with your doctor about any supplements you're considering before you start taking them — especially multivitamins that have a combination of micronutrients, as well as fat-soluble vitamins.

If you smoke, consider quitting smoking

While you may have heard of the negative effects of smoking throughout the entire body (including your skin), smoking has also been linked to hair loss..Overall, smoking may worsen hair loss because of its inflammatory effects in the body. ResearchersTrusted Source also believe that smoking can disrupt the growth cycle of your hair and even lead to color loss.

Try to reduce stress

While stress is a natural part of life, long-term stress can do damage to your health — including your hair. Researchers believe that cortisol, a stress hormone released by your adrenal glands, may disrupt your hair growth cycle..To help manage stress, it's important to take some time for yourself, whether it's a meditation session or a relaxing hobby you enjoy. You may also consider talking with a therapist if you're having a difficult time with chronic stress.

Take care of your hair

While you may be focused on reversing thinning hair, it's also important to try to practice good hair care techniques. Consider gentle hair products when available, and comb and brush hair only when needed. You can also place less stress on your hair by limiting the use of heated styling tools as well as tight hairstyles.

When to talk with a doctor about thinning hair

Although it's common to lose hair throughout the day, it's a good idea to speak with your doctor if you're losing more than 100 hairs per day. You should also talk with your doctor if you're worried about persistent hair loss or a receding hairline or if you notice sudden patchy hair loss. Patches of hair loss could signify an underlying medical condition.

CONCLUSION

Hair loss related to androgenic alopecia tends to happen gradually. While some people might experience hair loss as early as puberty, others might not notice symptoms until their middle ages. Female pattern baldness often results in thinning all over the scalp and might look like widening or thinning around the part. It typically occurs after age 65 but, for some females, it can begin early in their lives. Male pattern baldness typically involves progressive hair loss above the temples and thinning at the crown of the head, creating an "M" shape.